If You Practice SELF-LOVE You Will Never Spend A Day in Therapy

SELF-LOVE JOURNAL
ISBN Hardcover: 979-8-3482-2997-9
ISBN Paperback: 979-8-3482-3004-3

SELF-LOVE JOURNAL with 7-SHIFT PLANNER
ISBN Hardcover: 979-8-3482-3012-8
ISBN Paperback: 979-8-3482-3023-4

My Self-Love Notes
The Most Important Relationship Is the One You Have with Yourself
Self-Love Is a Daily Practice

"You Don't Find Love, You Create Love" Sharon Esther Lampert

My Self-Love Notes
The Most Important Relationship Is the One You Have with Yourself
Self-Love Is a Daily Practice

"You Don't Find Love, You Create Love" Sharon Esther Lampert

My Self-Love Notes
The Most Important Relationship Is the One You Have with Yourself
Self-Love Is a Daily Practice

"You Don't Find Love, You Create Love" Sharon Esther Lampert

My Self-Love Notes
The Most Important Relationship Is the One You Have with Yourself
Self-Love Is a Daily Practice

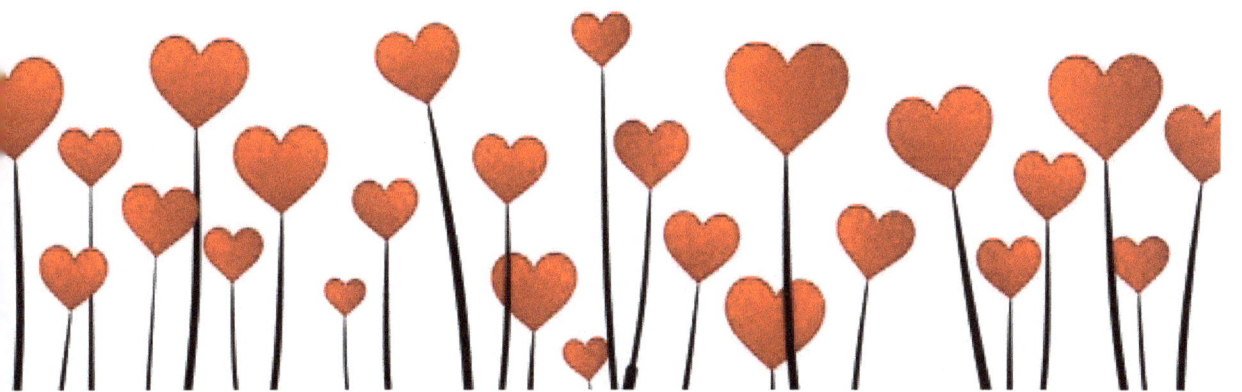

"You Don't Find Love, You Create Love" Sharon Esther Lampert

My Self-Love Notes
The Most Important Relationship Is the One You Have with Yourself
Self-Love Is a Daily Practice

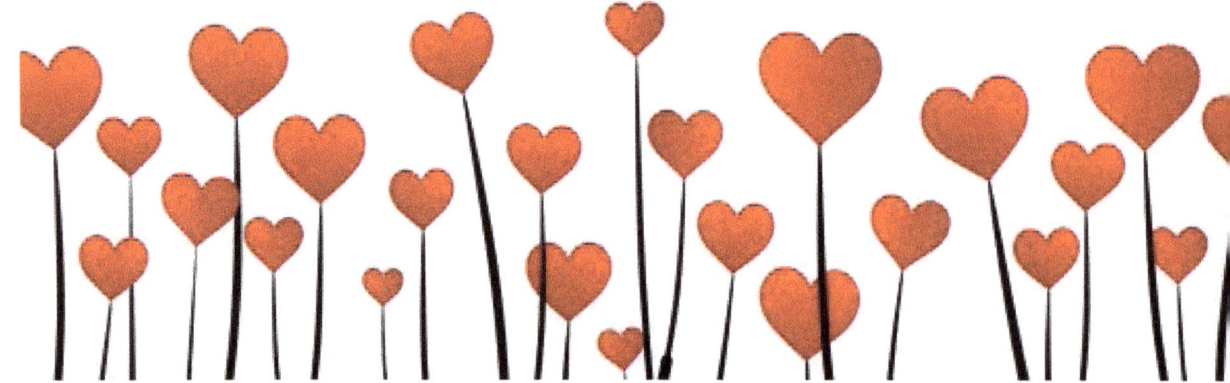

"You Don't Find Love, You Create Love" Sharon Esther Lampert

My Self-Love Notes
The Most Important Relationship Is the One You Have with Yourself
Self-Love Is a Daily Practice

"You Don't Find Love, You Create Love" Sharon Esther Lampert

My Self-Love Notes
The Most Important Relationship Is the One You Have with Yourself
Self-Love Is a Daily Practice

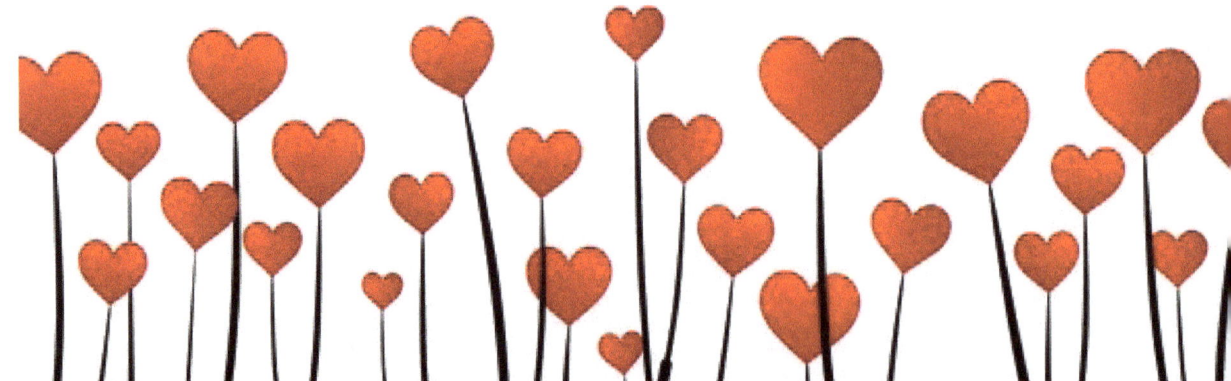

"You Don't Find Love, You Create Love" Sharon Esther Lampert

My Self-Love Notes
The Most Important Relationship Is the One You Have with Yourself
Self-Love Is a Daily Practice

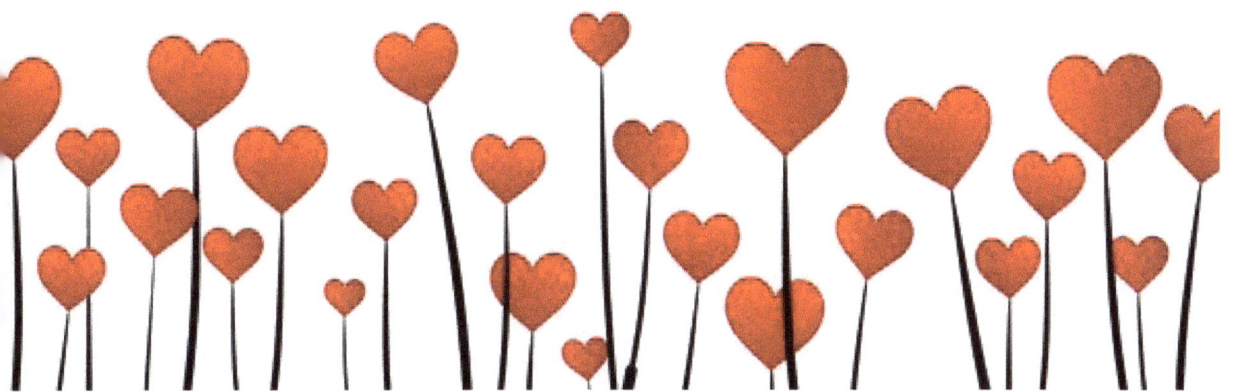

"You Don't Find Love, You Create Love" Sharon Esther Lampert

My Self-Love Notes
The Most Important Relationship Is the One You Have with Yourself
Self-Love Is a Daily Practice

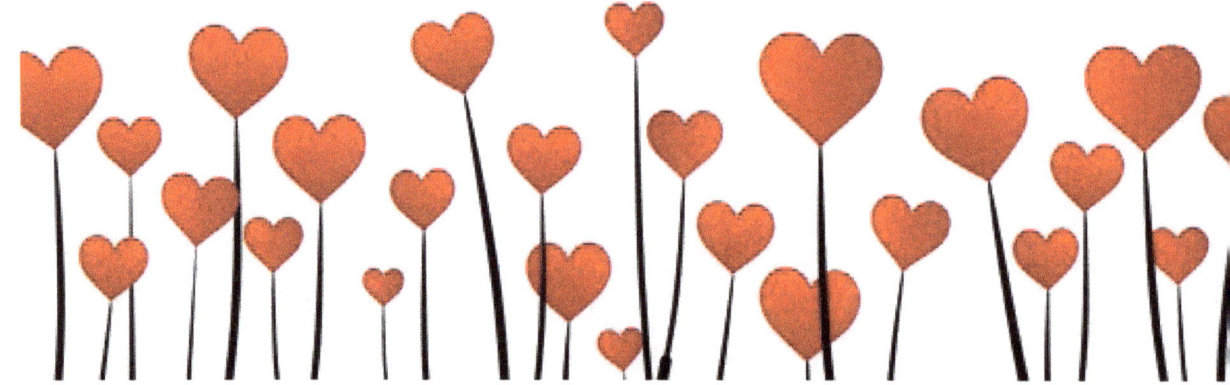

"You Don't Find Love, You Create Love" Sharon Esther Lampert

My Self-Love Notes
The Most Important Relationship Is the One You Have with Yourself
Self-Love Is a Daily Practice

"You Don't Find Love, You Create Love" Sharon Esther Lampert

My Self-Love Notes
The Most Important Relationship Is the One You Have with Yourself
Self-Love Is a Daily Practice

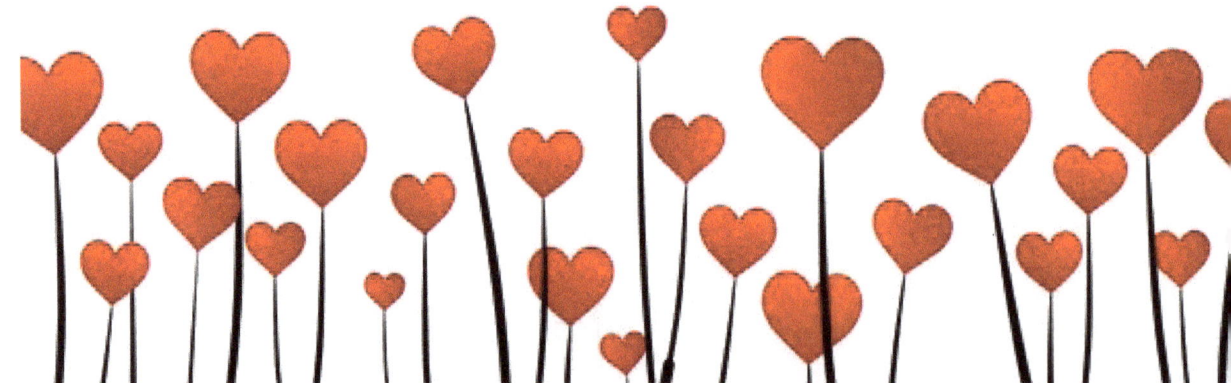

"You Don't Find Love, You Create Love" Sharon Esther Lampert

My Self-Love Notes
The Most Important Relationship Is the One You Have with Yourself
Self-Love Is a Daily Practice

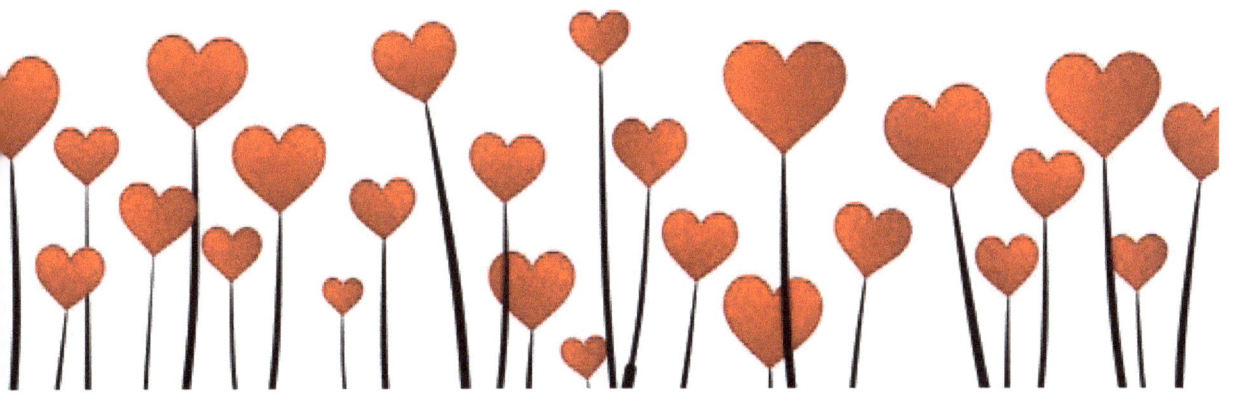

"You Don't Find Love, You Create Love" Sharon Esther Lampert

My Self-Love Notes
The Most Important Relationship Is the One You Have with Yourself
Self-Love Is a Daily Practice

"You Don't Find Love, You Create Love" Sharon Esther Lampert

My Self-Love Notes
The Most Important Relationship Is the One You Have with Yourself
Self-Love Is a Daily Practice

"You Don't Find Love. You Create Love" Sharon Esther Lampert

My Self-Love Notes
The Most Important Relationship Is the One You Have with Yourself
Self-Love Is a Daily Practice

"You Don't Find Love, You Create Love" Sharon Esther Lampert

My Self-Love Notes
The Most Important Relationship Is the One You Have with Yourself
Self-Love Is a Daily Practice

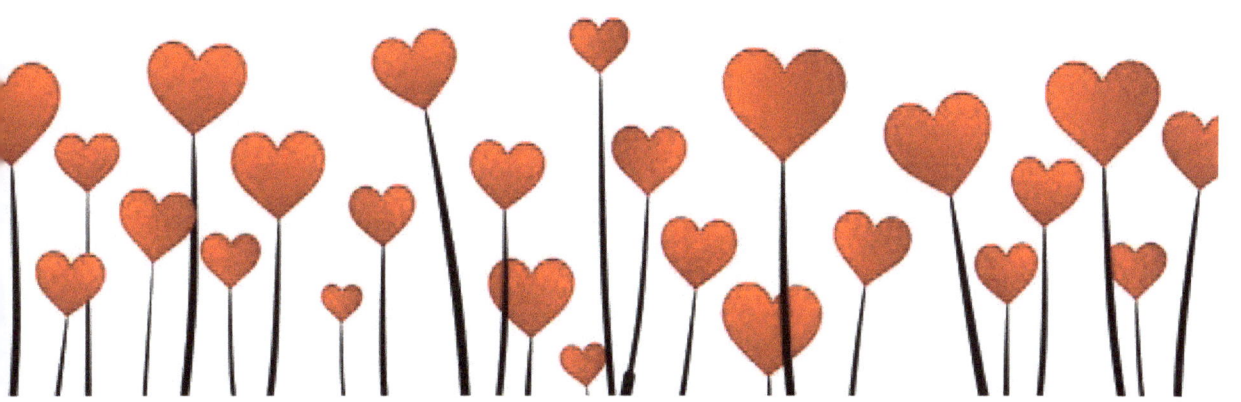

"You Don't Find Love, You Create Love" Sharon Esther Lampert

My Self-Love Notes
The Most Important Relationship Is the One You Have with Yourself
Self-Love Is a Daily Practice

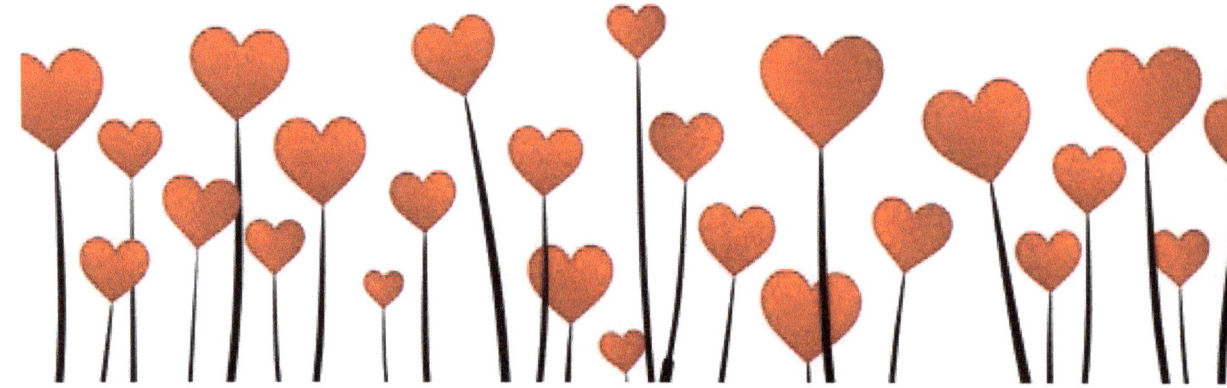

"You Don't Find Love, You Create Love" Sharon Esther Lampert

My Self-Love Notes
The Most Important Relationship Is the One You Have with Yourself
Self-Love Is a Daily Practice

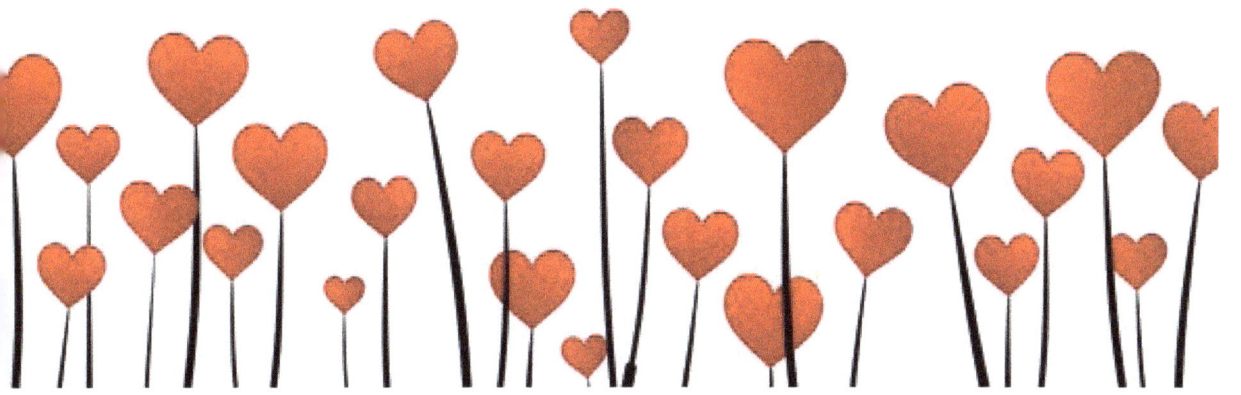

"You Don't Find Love. You Create Love" Sharon Esther Lampert

My Self-Love Notes
The Most Important Relationship Is the One You Have with Yourself
Self-Love Is a Daily Practice

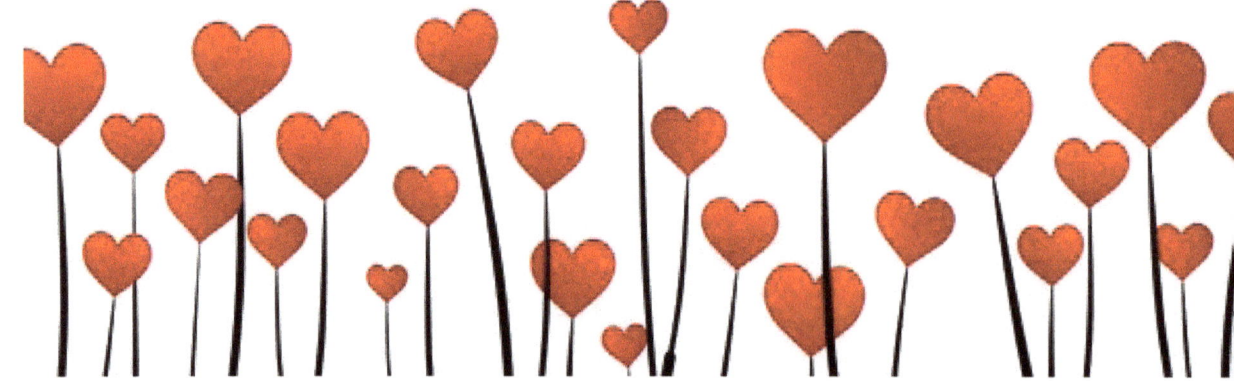

"You Don't Find Love, You Create Love" Sharon Esther Lampert

My Self-Love Notes
The Most Important Relationship Is the One You Have with Yourself
Self-Love Is a Daily Practice

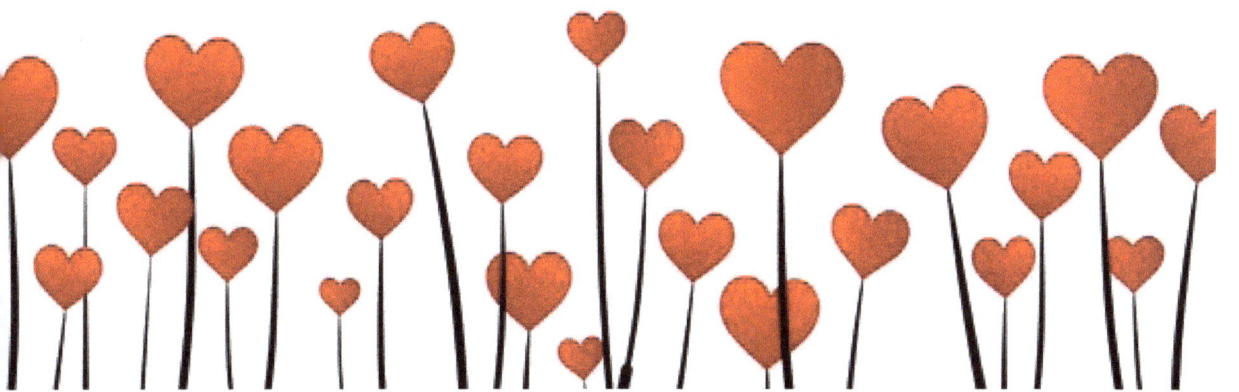

"You Don't Find Love, You Create Love" Sharon Esther Lampert

My Self-Love Notes
The Most Important Relationship Is the One You Have with Yourself
Self-Love Is a Daily Practice

"You Don't Find Love, You Create Love" Sharon Esther Lampert

My Self-Love Notes
The Most Important Relationship Is the One You Have with Yourself
Self-Love Is a Daily Practice

"You Don't Find Love, You Create Love" Sharon Esther Lampert

My Self-Love Notes
The Most Important Relationship Is the One You Have with Yourself
Self-Love Is a Daily Practice

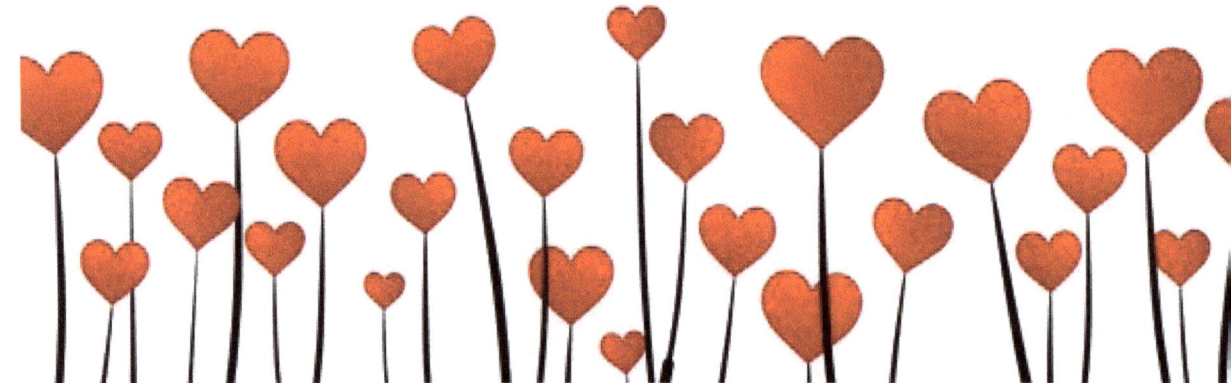

"You Don't Find Love, You Create Love" Sharon Esther Lampert

My Self-Love Notes
The Most Important Relationship Is the One You Have with Yourself
Self-Love Is a Daily Practice

"You Don't Find Love, You Create Love" Sharon Esther Lampert

My Self-Love Notes
The Most Important Relationship Is the One You Have with Yourself
Self-Love Is a Daily Practice

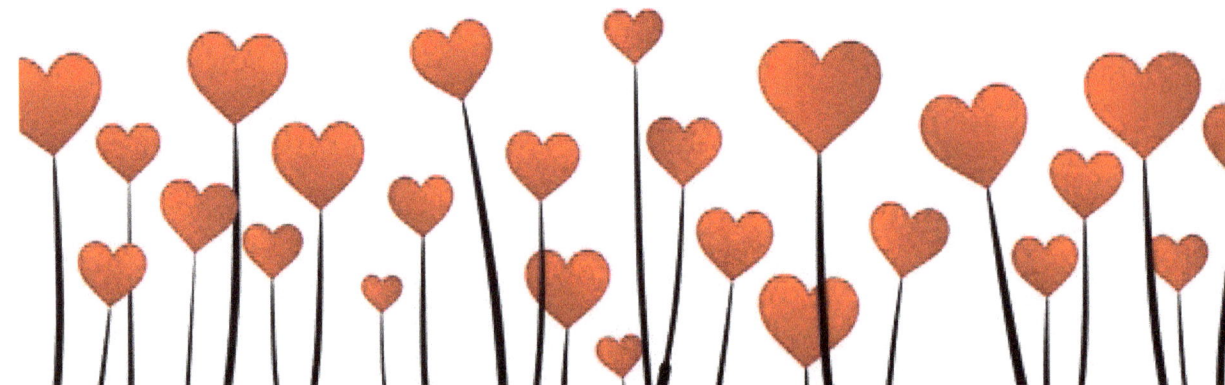

"You Don't Find Love, You Create Love" Sharon Esther Lampert

My Self-Love Notes
The Most Important Relationship Is the One You Have with Yourself
Self-Love Is a Daily Practice

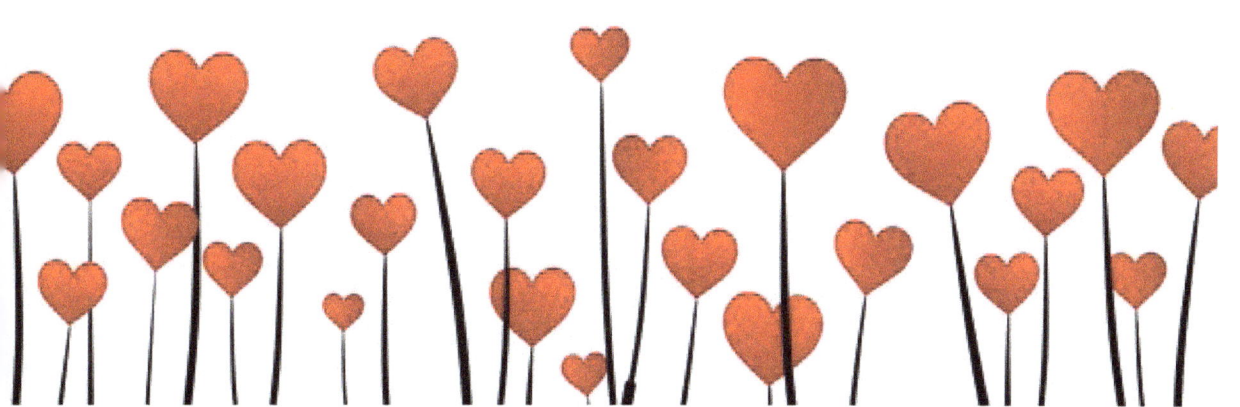

"You Don't Find Love, You Create Love" Sharon Esther Lampert

My Self-Love Notes
The Most Important Relationship Is the One You Have with Yourself
Self-Love Is a Daily Practice

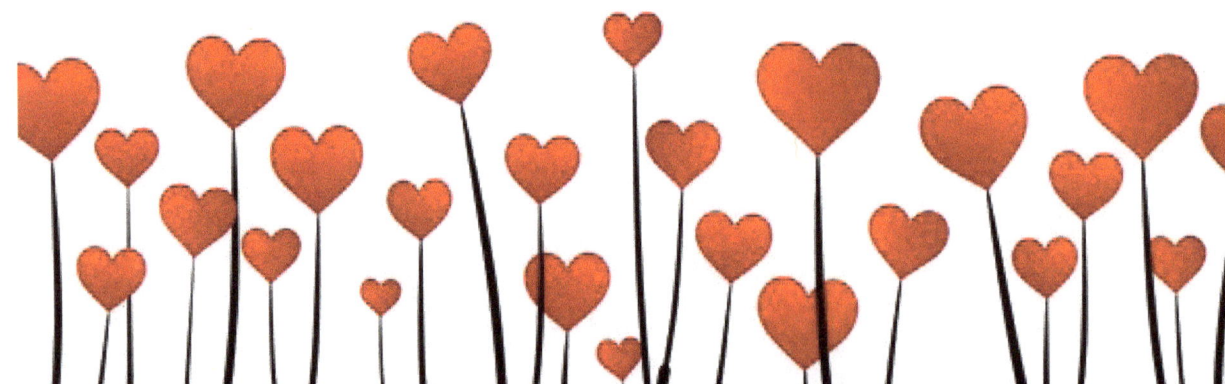

"You Don't Find Love, You Create Love" Sharon Esther Lampert

My Self-Love Notes
The Most Important Relationship Is the One You Have with Yourself
Self-Love Is a Daily Practice

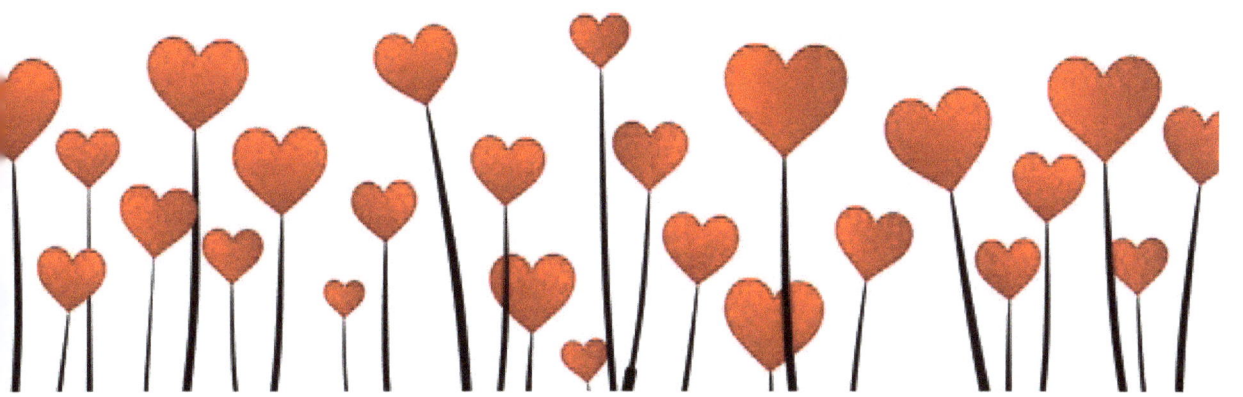

"You Don't Find Love, You Create Love" Sharon Esther Lampert

My Self-Love Notes
The Most Important Relationship Is the One You Have with Yourself
Self-Love Is a Daily Practice

"You Don't Find Love, You Create Love" Sharon Esther Lampert

My Self-Love Notes
The Most Important Relationship Is the One You Have with Yourself
Self-Love Is a Daily Practice

"You Don't Find Love, You Create Love" Sharon Esther Lampert

My Self-Love Notes
The Most Important Relationship Is the One You Have with Yourself
Self-Love Is a Daily Practice

"You Don't Find Love, You Create Love" Sharon Esther Lampert

My Self-Love Notes
The Most Important Relationship Is the One You Have with Yourself
Self-Love Is a Daily Practice

"You Don't Find Love, You Create Love" Sharon Esther Lampert

My Self-Love Notes
The Most Important Relationship Is the One You Have with Yourself
Self-Love Is a Daily Practice

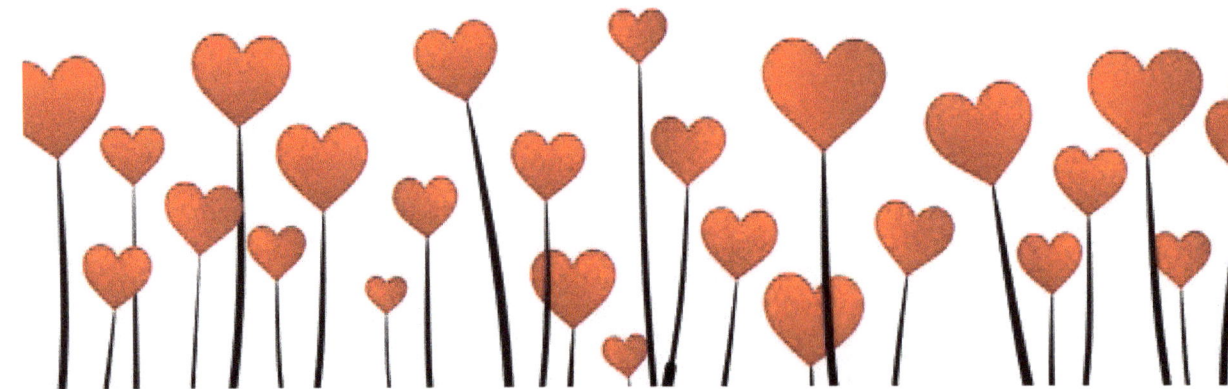

"You Don't Find Love, You Create Love" Sharon Esther Lampert

My Self-Love Notes
The Most Important Relationship Is the One You Have with Yourself
Self-Love Is a Daily Practice

"You Don't Find Love, You Create Love" Sharon Esther Lampert

My Self-Love Notes
The Most Important Relationship Is the One You Have with Yourself
Self-Love Is a Daily Practice

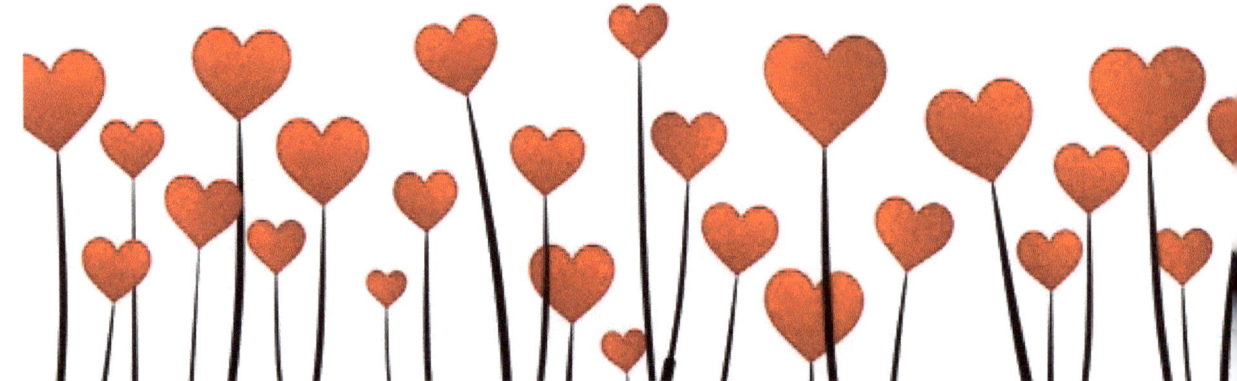

"You Don't Find Love, You Create Love" Sharon Esther Lampert

My Self-Love Notes
The Most Important Relationship Is the One You Have with Yourself
Self-Love Is a Daily Practice

"You Don't Find Love, You Create Love" Sharon Esther Lampert

My Self-Love Notes
The Most Important Relationship Is the One You Have with Yourself
Self-Love Is a Daily Practice

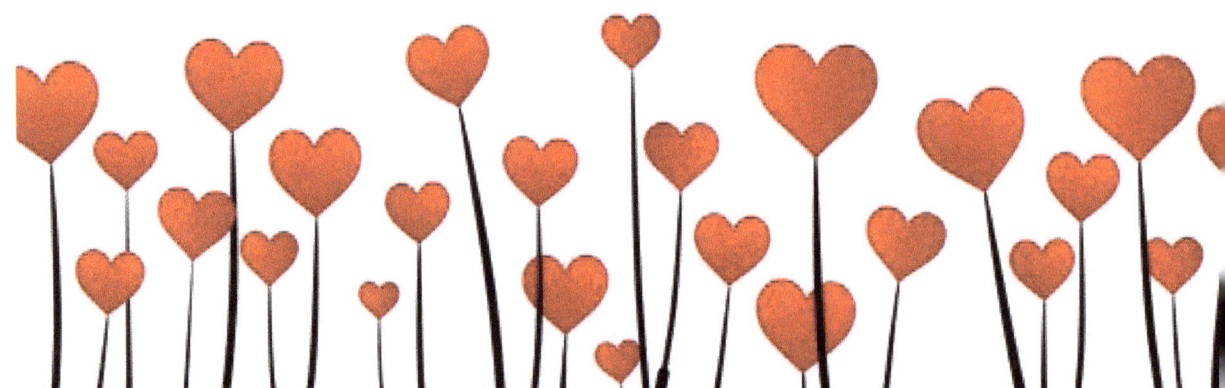

"You Don't Find Love, You Create Love" Sharon Esther Lampert

My Self-Love Notes
The Most Important Relationship Is the One You Have with Yourself
Self-Love Is a Daily Practice

"You Don't Find Love, You Create Love" Sharon Esther Lampert

My Self-Love Notes
The Most Important Relationship Is the One You Have with Yourself
Self-Love Is a Daily Practice

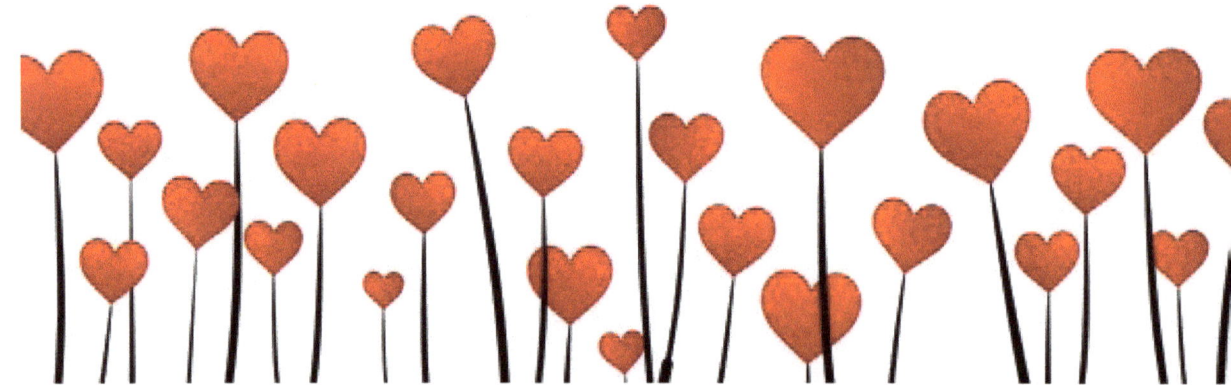

"You Don't Find Love, You Create Love" Sharon Esther Lampert

My Self-Love Notes
The Most Important Relationship Is the One You Have with Yourself
Self-Love Is a Daily Practice

"You Don't Find Love, You Create Love" Sharon Esther Lampert

My Self-Love Notes
The Most Important Relationship Is the One You Have with Yourself
Self-Love Is a Daily Practice

"You Don't Find Love, You Create Love" Sharon Esther Lampert

My Self-Love Notes
The Most Important Relationship Is the One You Have with Yourself
Self-Love Is a Daily Practice

"You Don't Find Love, You Create Love" Sharon Esther Lampert

My Self-Love Notes
The Most Important Relationship Is the One You Have with Yourself
Self-Love Is a Daily Practice

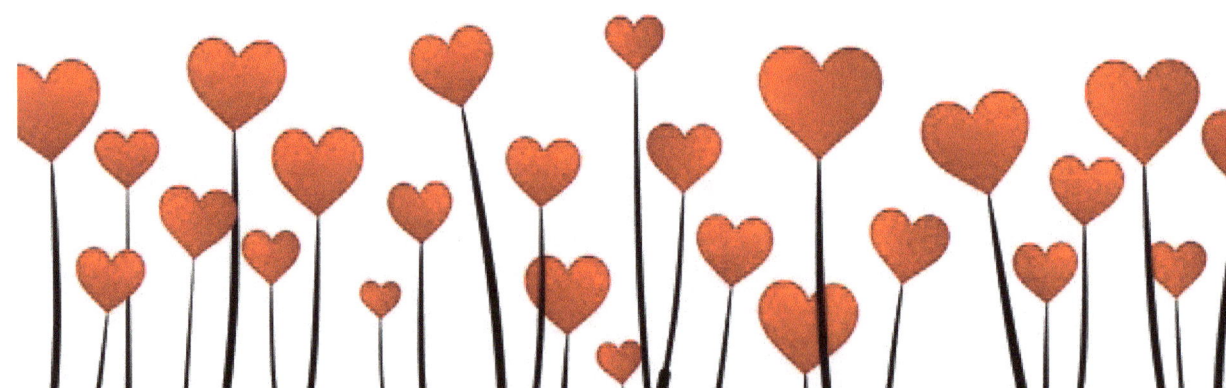

"You Don't Find Love, You Create Love" Sharon Esther Lampert

My Self-Love Notes
The Most Important Relationship Is the One You Have with Yourself
Self-Love Is a Daily Practice

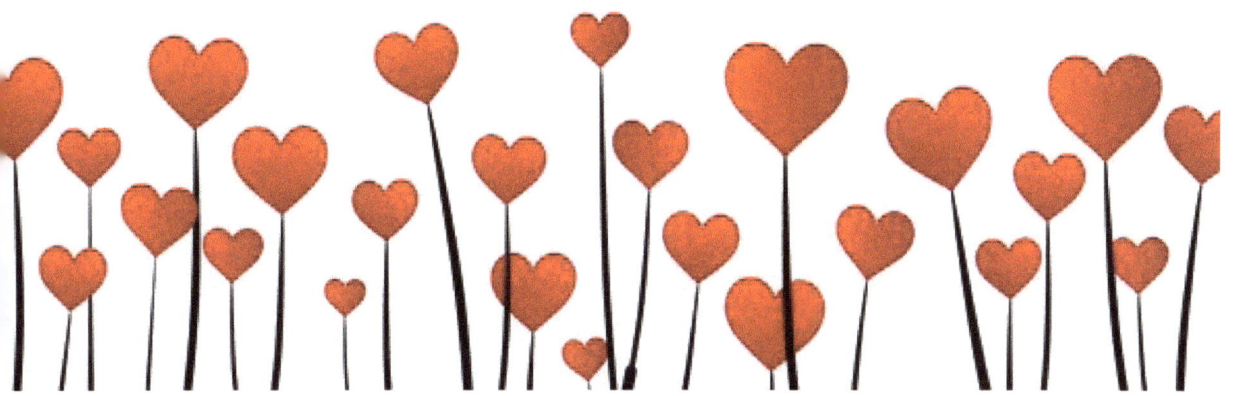

"You Don't Find Love, You Create Love" Sharon Esther Lampert

My Self-Love Notes
The Most Important Relationship Is the One You Have with Yourself
Self-Love Is a Daily Practice

"You Don't Find Love, You Create Love" Sharon Esther Lampert

My Self-Love Notes
The Most Important Relationship Is the One You Have with Yourself
Self-Love Is a Daily Practice

"You Don't Find Love, You Create Love" Sharon Esther Lampert

My Self-Love Notes
The Most Important Relationship Is the One You Have with Yourself
Self-Love Is a Daily Practice

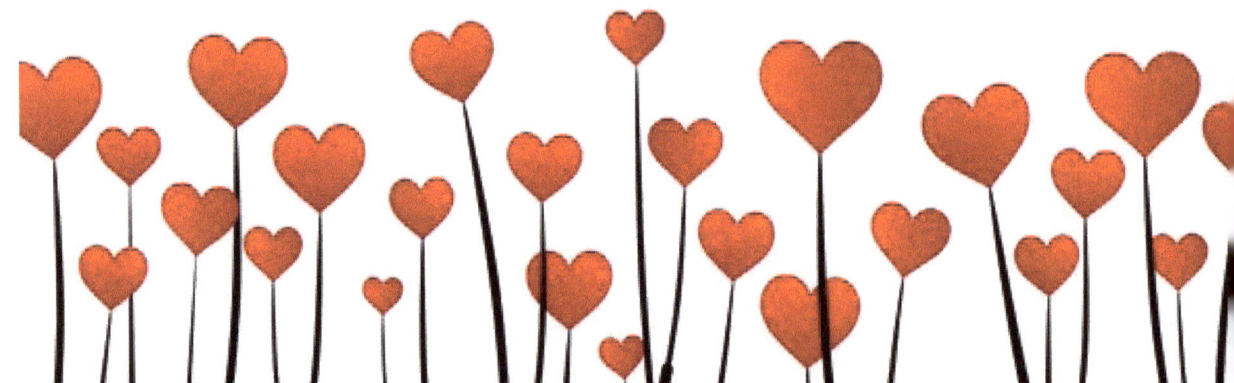

"You Don't Find Love, You Create Love" Sharon Esther Lampert

My Self-Love Notes
The Most Important Relationship Is the One You Have with Yourself
Self-Love Is a Daily Practice

"You Don't Find Love, You Create Love" Sharon Esther Lampert

My Self-Love Notes
The Most Important Relationship Is the One You Have with Yourself
Self-Love Is a Daily Practice

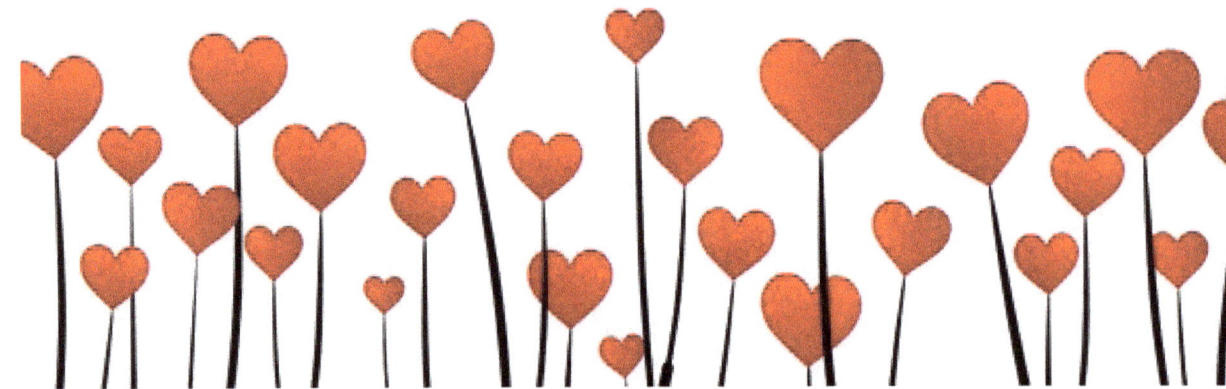

"You Don't Find Love, You Create Love" Sharon Esther Lampert

My Self-Love Notes
The Most Important Relationship Is the One You Have with Yourself
Self-Love Is a Daily Practice

"You Don't Find Love, You Create Love" Sharon Esther Lampert

My Self-Love Notes
The Most Important Relationship Is the One You Have with Yourself
Self-Love Is a Daily Practice

"You Don't Find Love, You Create Love" Sharon Esther Lampert

My Self-Love Notes
The Most Important Relationship Is the One You Have with Yourself
Self-Love Is a Daily Practice

"You Don't Find Love, You Create Love" Sharon Esther Lampert

My Self-Love Notes
The Most Important Relationship Is the One You Have with Yourself
Self-Love Is a Daily Practice

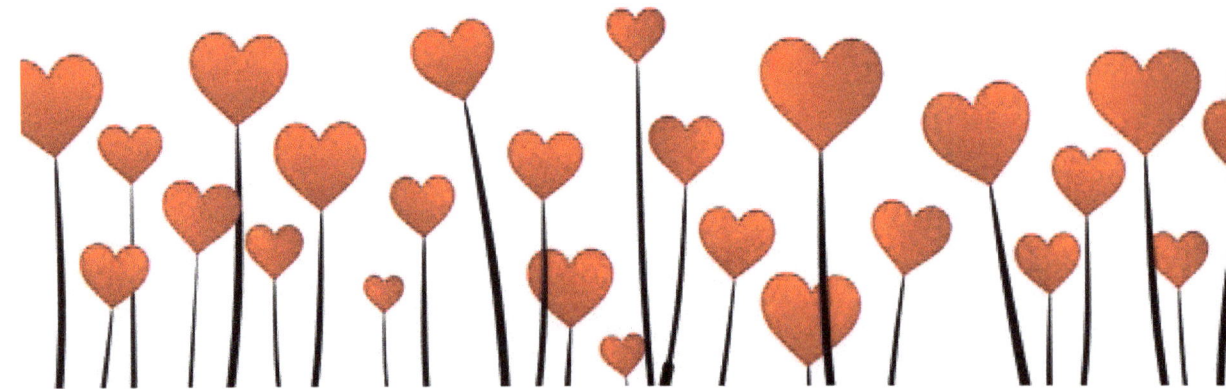

"You Don't Find Love, You Create Love" Sharon Esther Lampert

My Self-Love Notes
The Most Important Relationship Is the One You Have with Yourself
Self-Love Is a Daily Practice

"You Don't Find Love, You Create Love" Sharon Esther Lampert

My Self-Love Notes
The Most Important Relationship Is the One You Have with Yourself
Self-Love Is a Daily Practice

"You Don't Find Love, You Create Love" Sharon Esther Lampert

My Self-Love Notes
The Most Important Relationship Is the One You Have with Yourself
Self-Love Is a Daily Practice

"You Don't Find Love, You Create Love" Sharon Esther Lampert

My Self-Love Notes
The Most Important Relationship Is the One You Have with Yourself
Self-Love Is a Daily Practice

"You Don't Find Love, You Create Love" Sharon Esther Lampert

My Self-Love Notes
The Most Important Relationship Is the One You Have with Yourself
Self-Love Is a Daily Practice

"You Don't Find Love, You Create Love" Sharon Esther Lampert

My Self-Love Notes
The Most Important Relationship Is the One You Have with Yourself
Self-Love Is a Daily Practice

"You Don't Find Love, You Create Love" Sharon Esther Lampert

www.ingramcontent.com/pod-product-compliance
Lightning Source LLC
LaVergne TN
LVHW072121060526
838201LV00068B/4944